MW00440314

QUOTES FOR MEN

365 DAYS OF THE BEST INSPIRATIONAL QUOTES AND SAYINGS FOR MEN OF ALL AGES.

MICK KREMLING

Ó Copyright 2016 by Mick Kremling All rights reserved.

This document is geared towards providing exact and reliable information in regards to the topic and issue covered. The publication is sold with the idea that the publisher is not required to render accounting, officially permitted, or otherwise, qualified services. If advice is necessary, legal or professional, a practiced individual in the profession should be ordered.

From a Declaration of Principles which was accepted and approved equally by a Committee of the American Bar Association and a Committee of Publishers and Associations.

In no way is it legal to reproduce, duplicate, or transmit any part of this document in either electronic means or in printed format. Recording of this publication is strictly prohibited and any storage of this document is not allowed unless with written permission from the publisher. All rights reserved.

The information provided herein is stated to be truthful and consistent, in that any liability, in terms of inattention or otherwise, by any usage or abuse of any policies, processes, or directions contained within is the solitary and utter responsibility of the recipient reader. Under no circumstances will any legal responsibility or blame be held against the publisher for any reparation, damages, or monetary loss due to the information herein, either directly or indirectly.

Respective authors own all copyrights not held by the publisher.

The information herein is offered for informational purposes solely, and is universal as so. The presentation of the information is without contract or any type of guarantee assurance.

The trademarks that are used are without any consent, and the publication of the trademark is without permission or backing by the trademark owner. All trademarks and brands within this book are for clarifying purposes only and are the owned by the owners themselves, not affiliated with this document.

DAY 1

"SELF-CONTROL IS THE CHIEF ELEMENT IN SELF-RESPECT, AND SELF-RESPECT IS THE CHIEF ELEMENT IN COURAGE."

DAY 2

"THERE IS NOTHING IMPOSSIBLE TO HIM WHO WILL TRY."

-ALEXANDER THE GREAT

DAY 3

"THE LONGER I LIVE, THE MORE I AM CERTAIN THAT THE GREAT DIFFERENCE BETWEEN MEN, BETWEEN THE FEEBLE AND THE POWERFUL, THE GREAT AND INSIGNIFICANT- IS ENERGY, INVINCIBLE DETERMINATION. A PURPOSE ONCE FIXED AND THEN, VICTORY OR DEATH! THAT QUALITY WILL DO ANYTHING THAT CAN BE DONE IN THIS WORLD. NO TALENTS, NO CIRCUMSTANCES, NO OPPORTUNITIES, WILL MAKE A TWO LEGGED CREATURE A MAN WITHOUT IT."

- SIR THOMAS FOWELL BUXTON

DAY 4

"MEN ARE NOT BORN THEY ARE
CREATED. POVERTY, DIFFICULTY,
HEARTACHE, OPPRESSION, PAIN-
THESE ARE THE THINGS THAT
MAKE MEN OUT OF BOYS"

DAY 5

"IT IS THE BRAVE MAN'S PART TO
LIVE WITH GLORY, OR WITH
GLORY DIE."

-SOPHOCLES

DAY 6

"TO EVERY MAN UPON THIS
EARTH.

DEATH COMETH SOON OR LATE.

AND HOW CAN MAN DIE BETTER

THAN FACING FEARFUL ODDS,

FOR THE ASHES OF HIS FATHERS,

AND THE TEMPLES OF HIS GODS?"

DAY 7

"YOUR MIND WILL ANSWER MOST
QUESTIONS IF YOU LEARN TO
RELAX, AND WAIT FOR THE
ANSWER."

-WILLIAM S. BURROUGHS

DAY 8

FAR BETTER IS TO HAVE A STOUT
HEART ALWAYS AND SUFFER
ONE'S SHARE OF EVILS, THAN TO
BE EVER FEARING WHAT MAY
HAPPEN.

- HERODOTUS

DAY 9

BY TRAINING YOU WILL BE ABLE
TO FREELY CONTROL YOUR OWN
BODY, CONQUER MEN WITH YOUR
BODY, AND WITH SUFFICIENT
TRAINING YOU WILL BE ABLE TO
BEAT TEN MEN WITH YOUR
SPIRIT. WHEN YOU HAVE
REACHED THIS POINT, WILL IT
NOT MEAN THAT YOU ARE
INVINCIBLE?

DAY 10

"NOTHING HAPPENS TO ANY MAN
WHICH HE IS NOT FORMED BY
NATURE TO BEAR."

-MARCUS AURELIUS

DAY 11

"PERSEVERANCE, SECRET OF ALL TRIUMPHS"

-VICTOR HUGO

DAY 12

"STRENGTH, COURAGE, MASTERY, AND HONOR ARE THE *ALPHA* VIRTUES OF MEN ALL OVER THE WORLD. THEY ARE THE FUNDAMENTAL VIRTUES OF MEN BECAUSE WITHOUT THEM, NO 'HIGHER' VIRTUES CAN BE ENTERTAINED. YOU NEED TO BE ALIVE TO PHILOSOPHIZE. YOU CAN ADD TO THESE VIRTUES AND YOU CAN CREATE RULES AND MORAL CODES TO GOVERN THEM, BUT IF YOU REMOVE THEM FROM THE EQUATION ALTOGETHER YOU AREN'T JUST LEAVING BEHIND THE VIRTUES THAT ARE SPECIFIC

TO MEN, YOU ARE ABANDONING
THE VIRTUES THAT MAKE
CIVILIZATION POSSIBLE."

–JACK DONOVAN

DAY 13

"COURAGE IS NOT HAVING THE STRENGTH TO GO ON. IT IS GOING ON WHEN YOU DON'T HAVE THE STRENGTH."

DAY 14

"NO MAN HAS THE RIGHT TO BE AN AMATEUR IN THE MATTER OF PHYSICAL TRAINING. IT IS A SHAME FOR A MAN TO GROW OLD WITHOUT SEEING THE BEAUTY AND STRENGTH OF WHICH HIS BODY IS CAPABLE."

-SOCRATES

DAY 15

"THE WAY OF A SUPERIOR MAN IS
THREEFOLD: VIRTUOUS, HE IS
FREE FROM ANXIETIES; WISE, HE
IS FREE FROM PERPLEXITIES;
BOLD, HE IS FREE FROM FEAR."

–CONFUCIUS

DAY 16

"A WOMAN SIMPLY IS, BUT A MAN MUST BECOME. MASCUILITY IS RISKY AND ELUSIVE. IT IS ACHIEVED BY A REVOLT FROM WOMEN, AND IS CONFIRMED ONLY BY OTHER MEN. MANHOOD COERCED INTO SENSITIVITY IS NO MANHOOD AT ALL."

-CAMILLE PAGLIA

DAY 17

"IF YOU PUT A SMALL VALUE ON YOURSELF, REST ASSURED THE WORLD WILL NOT RAISE YOUR PRICE."

DAY 18

"DON'T WALK LIKE YOU RULE
THE WORLD, WALK LIKE YOU
DON'T CARE WHO DOES."

DAY 19

"WHEN YOU DIE, YOU WILL COME
FACE TO FACE WITH THE MAN
YOU COULD HAVE BECOME."

DAY 20

"IT IS BETTER TO STAND AND
FIGHT. IF YOU RUN, YOU'LL ONLY
DIE TIRED."

-VIKING SAYING

DAY 21

"STAND TRUE TO YOUR CALLING
TO BE A MAN. REAL WOMEN WILL
ALWAYS BE RELIEVED AND
GRATEFUL WHEN MEN ARE
WILLING TO BE MEN."

–Elisabeth Elliot

DAY 22

"THEY THAT CAN GIVE UP
ESSENTIAL LIBERTY TO
PURCHASE A LITTLE TEMPORARY
SAFETY, DESERVE NEITHER
LIBERTY NOR SAFETY."

-BEN FRANKLIN, 1759

DAY 23

"WORK UNTIL YOUR IDOLS BECOME YOUR RIVALS."

DAY 24

"THE SECRET OF CHANGE IS TO FOCUS ALL YOUR ENERGY, NOT ON FIGHTING THE OLD, BUT ON BUILDING THE NEW."

-SOCRATES

DAY 25

"IF YOU DO WHAT YOU ALWAYS DO, YOU WILL GET WHAT YOU ALWAYS GET.

DAY 26

"VICTORY IS RESERVED FOR THOSE WILLING TO PAY ITS PRICE."

-SUN TZU

DAY 27

LOVE YOUR PARENTS.

WE ARE OFTEN SO BUSY
GROWING UP THAT WE OFTEN
FORGET THEY ARE GROWING
OLD.

DAY 28

"IF A MAN DOES NOT STRIKE
FIRST, HE WILL BE FIRST
STRUCK."

- ATHENOGORAS OF SYRACUSE

DAY 29

"IT IS WELL THAT WAR IS SO
TERRIBLE, OR WE SHOULD GROW
TOO FOND OF IT."

ROBERT E. LEE

DAY 30

"EVERYTIME WE CHOOSE SAFETY,
WE REINFORCE FEAR."

-CHERI HUBER

DAY 45

"FIRST FIND THE MAN IN YOURSELF IF YOU WILL INSPIRE MANLINESS IN OTHERS."

-AMOS BRANSON ALCOTT

DAY 46

"THE MORE YOU KNOW,

THE LESS YOU NEED"

DAY 55

"BEFORE YOU ACT, LISTEN.
BEFORE YOU REACT, THINK.
BEFORE YOU SPEND, EARN.
BEFORE YOU CRITICIZE, WAIT.
BEFORE YOU PRAY, FORGIVE.
BEFORE YOU QUIT, TRY."

ERNEST HEMINGWAY

DAY 56

"OH, LOST TO VIRTUE- LOST TO
MANLY THOUGHT, LOST TO THE
NOBLE SALLIES OF THE SOUL!
WHO THINK IT SOLITUDE TO BE
ALONE."

-EDWARD YOUNG

DAY 57

"THERE COMES A CERTAIN POINT IN LIFE WHEN YOU HAVE TO STOP BLAMING OTHER PEOPLE FOR HOW YOU FEEL OR THE MISFORTUNES IN YOUR LIFE. YOU CAN'T GO THROUGH LIFE OBSESSING ABOUT WHAT MIGHT HAVE BEEN."

-HUGH JACKMAN

DAY 58

"I WILL EITHER FIND A WAY, OR
MAKE ONE"

- HANNIBAL BARCA

DAY 59

"WHEN A FATHER GIVES TO HIS
SON, BOTH LAUGH.

WHEN A SON GIVES TO HIS
FATHER, BOTH CRY."

-WILLIAM SHAKESPEARE

HE WHO, WITH STRONG PASSIONS, REMAINS CHASTE-HE WHO, KEENLY SENSITIVE, WITH MANLY POWER OF INDIGNATION IN HIM, CAN YET RESTRAIN HIMSELF AND FORGIVE- THESE ARE STRONG MEN, SPIRITUAL HEROES."

-FREDERICK WILLIAM ROBERTSON

DAY 61

"WHERE THERE IS NO STRUGGLE,
THERE IS NO STRENGTH."

DAY 62

"JUDGE YOUR SUCCESS BY WHAT
YOU GAVE UP IN ORDER TO
ACHIEVE IT."

- DALAI LAMA

DAY 63

"ADVERSITY TOUGHENS
MANHOOD, AND THE
CHARACTERISTIC OF THE GOOD
OR THE GREAT MAN IS NOT THAT
HE HAS BEEN EXEMPT FROM THE
EVILS OF LIFE, BUT THAT HE HAS
SURMOUNTED THEM."

-PATRICK HENRY

DAY 64

"IT'S BETTER TO KNOW AND BE
DISAPPOINTED THAN TO NEVER
KNOW AND ALWAYS WONDER."

DAY 65

"GO OFTEN TO THE HOUSE OF THY FRIEND, FOR WEEDS SOON CHOKE UP THE UNUSED PATH."

-CHINESE PROVERB

DAY 66

"LESSONS IN LIFE WILL BE
REPEATED UNTIL THEY ARE
LEARNED."

-FRANK SONNENBERG

DAY 67

"YOUR HEALTH ACCOUNT, YOUR BANK ACCOUNT, THEY'RE THE SAME THING. THE MORE YOU PUT IN, THE MORE YOU CAN TAKE OUT. EXERCISE IS KING AND NUTRITION IS QUEEN. TOGETHER YOU HAVE A KINGDOM."

-JACK LALANNE

DAY 68

"THERE IS A DIFFERENCE
BETWEEN BEING A GOOD MAN
AND BEING GOOD AT BEING A
MAN:

-JACK DONOVAN

DAY 69

"GOOD FELLOWSHIP AND
FRIENDSHIP ARE LASTING,
RATIONAL AND MANLY
PLEASURES."

-WILLIAM WYCHERLEY

DAY 70

"LET US RETURN TO A TIME WHEN
MEN WANTED TO PUT HAIR ON
THEIR CHEST, NOT TAKE IF OFF."

-THE BRATTENDER

DAY 71

LEADERSHIP IS A POTENT
COMBINATION OF STRATEGY AND
CHARACTER. BUT IF YOU MUST
BE WITHOUT ONE, BE WITHOUT
THE STRATEGY.

-NORMAN SCHWARZKOPF

DAY 72

"WHEN YOU WANT TO SUCCEED
AS BAD AS YOU WANT TO
BREATHE, THEN YOU WILL BE
SUCCESSFUL."

-Eric Thomas

DAY 73

"ALL IT TAKES FOR EVIL TO
SUCCEED IS FOR GOOD MEN TO
DO NOTHING."

~EDMUND BURKE

DAY 74

"A MAN WHO DARES TO WASTE
AN HOUR OF TIME HAS NOT
DISCOVERED THE VALUE OF
LIFE."

-CHARLES DARWIN

DAY 75

"IT IS NEVER TOO LATE TO BE WHAT YOU MIGHT HAVE BEEN"

GEORGE ELIOT

DAY 76

"YOUR BODY IS A GIFT. BE
THANKFUL FOR IT AND TREAT IT
WELL."

DAY 77

"WHY CHOOSE FAILURE WHEN SUCCESS IS AN OPTION?"

DAY 78

"WHAT WOULD YOU ATTEMPT TO DO IF YOU KNEW YOU COULD NOT FAIL?"

DAY 79

"THE GREATEST PLEASURE IN
LIFE IS DOING WHAT PEOPLE SAY
YOU CAN NOT DO."

DAY 80

"WE MUST EMBRACE PAIN AND BURN IT AS FUEL FOR OUR JOURNEY"

-KENJI MIYAZAWA

DAY 81

"NOTHING WILL WORK UNLESS
YOU DO."

-JOHN WOODEN

DAY 82

"RISE ABOVE HATE, PAIN, DEPRESSION, THE PAST."

DAY 83

EVERY FATHER SHOULD
REMEMBER THAT ONE DAY HIS
SON WILL FOLLOW HIS EXAMPLE,
NOT HIS ADVICE.

DAY 84

"YESTERDAY I WAS CLEVER, SO I
WANTED TO CHANGE THE WORLD.
TODAY I AM WISE, SO I AM
CHANGING MYSELF."

-RUMI

DAY 85

"I AM INDEED A KING, BECAUSE I
KNOW HOW TO RULE MYSELF."

-PIETRO ARETINO

DAY 86

"MAN SHOULD NOT ASK WHAT
THE MEANING OF HIS LIFE IS, BUT
RATHER MUST RECOGNIZE THAT
IT IS HE WHO IS ASKED."

-VIKTOR FRANKL

DAY 87

"MANY A BOOK IS LIKE A KEY TO AN UNKNOWN CHAMBER WITHIN THE CASTLE OF ONE'S OWN SELF."

-FRANZ KAFKA

DAY 88

THE HOUR IS FAST APPROACHING, ON WHICH THE HONOR AND SUCCESS OF THIS ARMY AND THE SAFETY OF OUR BLEEDING COUNTRY DEPEND. REMEMBER OFFICERS AND SOLDIERS, THAT YOU ARE FREE MEN, FIGHTING FOR THE BLESSINGS OF LIBERTY — THAT SLAVERY WILL BE YOUR PORTION, AND THAT OF YOUR POSTERITY, IF YOU DO NOT ACQUIT YOURSELVES LIKE MEN."

-GEORGE WASHINGTON, 1776

DAY 89

"ONE CANNOT ALWAYS BE A HERO, BUT ONE CAN ALWAYS BE A MAN."

-JOHANN WOLFGANG

DAY 90

"LOVE THY ART, POOR AS IT MAY BE, WHICH THOU HAST LEARNED, AND BE CONTENT WITH IT. PASS THROUGH THE REST OF LIKE ONE WHO HAS INTRUSTED TO THE GODS WITH HIS WHOLE SOUL ALL THAT HE HAS, MAKING THEYSELF NEITHER THE TYRANT NOR THE SLAVE OF ANY MAN."

-MARCUS AURELIUS

DAY 91

"FALL SEVEN TIMES, STAND UP EIGHT."

-JAPANESE PROVERB

DAY 92

"YOU DON'T DROWN BY FALLING
IN WATER, YOU DROWN BY
STAYING THERE."

DAY 93

"HE UNDERSTOOD WELL ENOUGH
HOW A MAN WITH A CHOICE
BETWEEN PRIDE AND
RESPONSIBILITY WILL ALMOST
ALWAYS CHOOSE PRIDE- IF
RESPONSIBILITY ROBS HIM OF HIS
MANHOOD."

-STEPHEN KING

DAY 94

FATHER:

A SON'S FIRST HERO

A DAUGHTER'S FIRST LOVE

DAY 95

"CIVILIZE THE MIND, BUT MAKE THE BODY SAVAGE."

DAY 96

"COURAGE IS NOT THE ABSENCE
OF FEAR, IT IS THE ABILITY TO
ACT IN THE PRESENCE OF FEAR."

DAY 97

"DO WHAT THY MANHOOD BIDS THEE DO, FROM NONE BUT SELF EXPECT APPLAUSE. HE NOBLEST LIVES AND NOBLEST DIES WHO MAKES AND KEEPS HIS SELF-MADE LAWS."

-RICHARD FRANCIS BURTON

DAY 98

FATE WHISPERED TO THE
WARRIOR

"YOU CANNOT DEFEAT THE
STORM"

THE WARRIOR WHISPERED BACK

"I AM THE STORM"

DAY 99

A BRAVE MAN MAY FALL, BUT HE CANNOT YIELD.

- LATIN PROVERB

DAY 100

"THIS IS YOUR WORLD. SHAPE IT
OR SOMEONE ELSE WILL."

DAY 101

"IMPOSSIBLE IS A WORD ONLY TO BE FOUND IN THE DICTIONARY OF FOOLS."

-NAPOLEON BONAPARTE

DAY 102

"TAKE RISKS, IF YOU WIN YOU'LL BE HAPPY. IF YOU LOSE, YOU'LL BE WISE.

DAY 103

"THERE IS NOTHING NOBLE IN
BEING SUPERIOR TO YOUR
FELLOW MAN; TRUE NOBILITY IS
BEING SUPERIOR TO YOUR
FORMER SELF."

-ERNEST HEMINGWAY

DAY 104

"IT'S NOT THE SIZE OF THE DOG IN THE FIGHT, IT'S THE SIZE OF THE FIGHT IN THE DOG."

-MARK TWAIN

DAY 105

"YOU DREAM. YOU PLAN. YOU REACH. THERE WILL BE OBSTACLES. THERE WILL BE DOUBTERS. THERE WILL BE MISTAKES. BUT WITH HARD WORK, WITH BELIEF, WITH CONFIDENCE AND TRUST IN YOURSELF AND THOSE AROUND YOU, THERE ARE NO LIMITS."

-MICHAEL PHELPS

DAY 106

"IT IS BETTER TO LIVE ONE DAY
AS A LION THAN A HUNDRED
YEARS AS A SHEEP.

-ROMAN PROVERB

DAY 107

"COWARDS DIE MANY TIMES BEFORE THEY DIE. THE VALIENT NEVER TASTE DEATH BUT ONCE."

-W. SHAKESPEARE

DAY 108

"MAN WAS ONCE WILD. DON'T LET THEM TAME YOU."

DAY 109

"DISCIPLINE, IS JUST CHOOSING BETWEEN WHAT YOU WANT NOW, AND WHAT YOU WANT MOST."

DAY 110

"MAY YOUR PASSION BE THE
KERNEL OF CORN STUCK
BETWEEN YOUR TEETH, ALWAYS
REMINDING YOU THERE IS
SOMETHING TO ATTEND TO."

-JEB DICKERSON

DAY 111

"YOUR TASK WILL NOT BE AN
EASY ONE. YOUR ENEMY IS WELL
TRAINED, WELL EQUIPPED AND
BATTLE HARDENED. HE WILL
FIGHT SAVAGELY"

**GENERAL DWIGHT D. EISENHOWER – 6
JUNE 1944**

DAY 112

"SCAR TISSUE IS STRONGER THAN REGULAR TISSUE. REALIZE THE STRENGTH, MOVE ON.

-HENRY ROLLINS

DAY 113

"THE WOLF ON TOP THE HILL IS NEVER AS HUNGRY AS THE WOLF CLIMBING UP THE HILL"

DAY 114

"REALIZE DEEPLY THAT THE
PRESENT MOMENT IS ALL YOU
EVER HAVE."

DAY 115

"HE WHO ASKS A QUESTION IS A FOOL FOR A MINUTE; HE WHO DOES NOT REMAINS A FOOL FOREVER."

-CHINESE PROVERB

DAY 116

THERE IS NOW NO HOPE OF
ESCAPING. IF YOU FIGHT YOU
WILL CONQUER, BUT IF YOU FLEE
YOU WILL FALL.

- FULCHER OF CHARTRES

DAY 117

"IN THE END WHAT SEPARATES A
MAN FROM A SLAVE? MONEY?
POWER? NO, A MAN CHOOSES,
AND A SLAVE OBEYS!

-ANDREW RYAN

DAY 118

DANGER GLEAMS LIKE SUNSHINE
TO A BRAVE MAN'S EYES.

- EURIPIDES

DAY 119

"WE SLEEP SAFE IN OUR BEDS
BECAUSE ROUGH MEN STAND
READY IN THE NIGHT TO VISIT
VIOLENCE ON THOSE WHO
WOULD DO US HARM."

-GEORGE ORWELL

DAY 120

"BE SURE TO TASTE YOUR WORDS
BEFORE YOU SPIT THEM OUT."

DAY 121

"IT NEVER GETS EASIER. YOU JUST GET STRONGER."

DAY 122

"BE THE TYPE OF PERSON YOU WANT TO MEET."

DAY 123

"MAKE THYSELF A CRAFTSMAN IN SPEECH, FOR THEREBY THOU SHALT GAIN THE UPPERHAND."

-INSCRIPTION FOUND IN A 5,000 YEAR OLD EGYPTIAN TOMB

DAY 124

"THE LION DOES NOT CONCERN ITSELF WITH THE OPINIONS OF SHEEP."

DAY 125

THE SPARTANS DO NOT ASK HOW MANY, BUT WHERE THEY ARE.

KING AGIS II OF SPARTA, 427 BC

DAY 126

"I'M STRONGER BECAUSE I HAD
TO BE, I'M SMARTER BECAUSE OF
MY MISTAKES, HAPPIER BECAUSE
OF THE SADNESS I'VE KNOWN,
AND NOW WISER BECAUSE I
LEARNED."

DAY 127

"YOU CAN TELL THE GREATNESS
OF A MAN BY WHAT MAKES HIM
ANGRY"

DAY 128

"THERE ARE ONLY TWO OPTIONS, MAKE PROGRESS OR MAKE EXCUSES"

DAY 129

"THE WORK GOES ON, THE CAUSE
ENDURES, THE HOPE STILL LIVES,
AND THE DREAMS SHALL NEVER
DIE"

-TED KENNEDY

DAY 130

"IF YOU WANT SOMETHING
YOU'VE NEVER HAD, THEN YOU
MUST DO SOMETHING YOU'VE
NEVER DONE."

DAY 131

"THE WORLD MAKES WAY FOR
THE MAN WHO KNOWS WHERE HE
IS GOING."

-RALPH WALDO EMERSON

DAY 132

"A CONSTANT STRUGGLE, A CEASELESS BATTLE TO BRING SUCCESS FROM INHOSPITABLE SURROUNDINGS, IS THE PRICE FOR ALL GREAT ACHIEVEMENTS."

-ORISON SWETT MARDEN

DAY 133

"WHAT YOU LEAVE BEHIND IS NOT THAT WHICH IS ENGRAVED IN STONE MONUMENTS, BUT THAT WHICH IS WOVEN INTO THE LIVES OF OTHERS."

-PERICLES

DAY 134

"YOU MUST SHOW NO MERCY...
NOR HAVE ANY BELIEF
WHATSOEVER IN HOW OTHERS
JUDGE YOU...FOR YOUR
GREATNESS WILL SILENCE THEM
ALL."

-UNKNOWN WARRIOR

DAY 135

"YOU WILL NOT BE PUNISHED FOR YOUR ANGER; YOU WILL BE PUNISHED BY YOUR ANGER."

DAY 136

"NO MAN IS MORE UNHAPPY
THAN HE WHO NEVER FACES
ADVERSITY. FOR HE IS NOT
PERMITTED TO PROVE HIMSELF."

-SENECA

DAY 137

"A FIRM TREE DOES NOT FEAR
THE STORM."

DAY 138

"SHOW ME THE MAN YOU HONOR, AND I WILL KNOW WHAT KIND OF A MAN YOU ARE, FOR IT SHOWS ME WHAT YOUR IDEAL OF MANHOOD IS, AND WHAT KIND OF A MAN YOU LONG TO BE."

-THOMAS CARLYLE

DAY 139

TO THOSE THAT FLEE COMES

NEITHER POWER NOR GLORY

- HOMER

DAY 140

WHEN YOU TEACH YOUR SON,
YOU TEACH YOUR SON'S SON.

DAY 141

"THE MORE COMFORT THE LESS COURAGE THERE IS."

-FIELD MARSHAL PRINCE ALEKSANDR V. SUVOROV

DAY 142

"THE STRONG DO WHAT THEY CAN.

THE WEAK SUFFER WHAT THEY MUST."

DAY 143

"ALWAYS FORGIVE YOUR
ENEMIES - NOTHING ANNOYS
THEM SO MUCH."

-OSCAR WILDE

DAY 144

"WISE MEN SPEAK BECAUSE THEY
HAVE SOMETHING TO SAY, FOOLS
SPEAK BECAUSE THEY HAVE TO
SAY SOMETHING."

-PLATO

DAY 145

"A MAN'S LEDGER DOES NOT
TELL WHAT HE IS OR WHAT HE'S
WORTH. COUNT WHAT IS IN MAN,
NOT WHAT IS ON HIM, IF YOU
WOULD KNOW WHAT HE IS
WORTH, WHETHER RICH OR
POOR."

-HENRY WARD BEECHER

DAY 146

"THE DISADVANTAGE OF
BECOMING WISE IS TO REALIZE
HOW FOOLISH YOU'VE BEEN."

-EVAN ESAR

DAY 147

"YOU WILL NEVER COME UP
AGAINST A GREATER ADVERSARY
THAN YOUR OWN POTENTIAL"

DAY 148

"THERE ARE TWO THINGS A MAN
SHOULD NEVER BE ANGRY AT,
WHAT HE CAN HELP, AND WHAT
HE CAN NOT."

-PLATO

DAY 149

"SUFFER THE PAIN OF DISCIPLINE OR SUFFER THE PAIN OF REGRET"

DAY 150

"FORMAL EDUCATION WILL MAKE
YOU A LIVING. SELF-EDUCATION
WILL MAKE YOU A FORTUNE."

DAY 151

"REMEMBER THAT GUY THAT
GAVE UP? NEITHER DOES
ANYBODY ELSE."

DAY 152

"MAY WE EVER CHOOSE THE
HARDER RIGHT, INSTEAD OF THE
EARLIER WRONG."

-THOMAS S. MONSON

DAY 153

"AN INVASION OF ARMIES CAN BE RESISTED, BUT NOT AN IDEA WHOSE TIME HAS COME."

-VICTOR HUGO

DAY 154

"THE GREATEST GLORY IN LIVING
LIES NOT IN NEVER FAILING, BUT
IN RISING EVERYTIME WE FALL.

-NELSON MANDELA

DAY 155

"BLESSED IS HE WHO EXPECTS
NOTHING, FOR HE SHALL NEVER
BE DISAPPOINTED."

-ALEXANDER POPE

DAY 156

"DO NOT PRAY FOR AN EASY LIFE.
PRAY FOR THE STRENGTH TO
ENDURE A DIFFICULT ONE."

-BRUCE LEE

DAY 157

"ASKING FOR THE TRUTH DOES NOT MAKE A MAN A FOOL, BUT BELIEVING THE ANSWER DOES."

-BRYNNER FOX

DAY 158

"OPPORTUNITY IS MISSED BY
MOST MEN BECAUSE IT IS
DRESSED IN OVERALLS AND
LOOKS LIKE WORK."

-THOMAS EDISON

DAY 159

"IMPOSSIBLE IS POTENTIAL.
IMPOSSIBLE IS TEMPORARY.
IMPOSSIBLE IS NOTHING."

-MUHAMMAD ALI

DAY 160

"YOU MAY ABANDON YOUR OWN BODY BUT YOU MUST PRESERVE YOUR HONOUR."

-MIYAMOTO MUSASHI

DAY 161

"A MAN IS ONE WHOSE BODY HAS BEEN TRAINED TO BE THE READY SERVANT OF HIS MIND, WHOSE PASSIONS ARE TRAINED TO BE THE SERVANTS OF HIS WILL, WHO ENJOYS THE BEAUTIFUL, LOVES TRUTH, HATES WRONG, LOVES TO DO GOOD, AND RESPECTS OTHERS AS HIMSELF."

-JOHN RUSKIN

DAY 162

"THE BEST PLACE TO FIND A
HELPING HAND IS AT THE END OF
YOUR OWN ARM."

-SWEDISH PROVERB

DAY 163

"WITHOUT AN ADVERSARY, VIRTUE SHRIVELS. WE SEE HOW GREAT AND HOW VIABLE VIRTUE IS WHEN, BY ENDURANCE, IT SHOWS WHAT IT IS CAPABLE OF."

-SENECA

DAY 164

"A SUCCESSFUL MAN IS HE WHO BUILDS A FOUNDATION WITH THE BRICKS OTHERS HAVE THROWN AT HIM."

-DAVID BRINKLEY

DAY 165

"THE GREATEST WEALTH IS A
POVERTY OF DESIRES"

-SENECA

DAY 166

"THOSE MEN GET ALONG BEST WITH WOMEN WHO GET ALONG BEST WITHOUT THEM"

DAY 167

"BEGIN-TO BEGIN IS HALF THE
WORK, LET HALF STILL REMAIN,
AGAIN BEGIN THIS, AND THOU
WILT HAVE FINISHED!"

-MARCUS AURELIUS

DAY 168

"VALOUR IS THE CONTEMPT OF
DEATH AND PAIN."

- TACITUS

DAY 169

"IF OPPORTUNITY DOESN'T KNOCK, BUILD A DOOR."

-DALAI LAMA

DAY 170

"THE COURAGE WE DESIRE AND
PRIZE IS NOT THE COURAGE TO
DIE DECENTLY, BUT TO LIVE
MANFULLY."

-THOMAS CARLYLE

"MEN HAVE DISCOVERED THEIR DISTICTIVE VIRTUES AND VICES THROUGH GRAPPLING WITH THE PERENNIAL DILEMMAS AND DEMANDS OF LOVE, COURAGE, PRIDE, FAMILY, AND COUNTRY-THE FIVE PATHS WHOSE PROER ORDERING GIVES US THE KEY TO THE SECRET OF HAPPINESS FOR A MAN."

-WALLER NEWELL

"A MAN IS BORN GENTLE AND
WEAK. AT DEATH, HE IS HARD
AND STIFF. GREEN PLANTS ARE
TENDER AND FILLED WITH SAP.
AT DEATH, THEY ARE WITHERED
AND DRY. THEREFORE, THE STIFF
AND UNBENDING IS THE DISCIPLE
OF DEATH, AND THE GENTLE AND
YIELDING IS THE DISCIPLE OF
LIFE."

-LAO TZU

DAY 173

"FOR THE MAN WHO MAKES EVERYTHING THAT LEADS TO HAPPINESS, OR NEAR TO IT, TO DEPEND UPON HIMSELF, AND NOT UPON OTHER MEN...HAS ADOPTED THE VERY BEST PLAN FOR LIVING HAPPILY. THIS IS THE MAN OF MODERATION; THIS IS THE MAN OF MANLY CHARACTER AND OF WISDOM."

-PLATO

DAY 174

"THE TEST OF EVERY RELIGIOUS,
POLITCAL, OR EDUCATIONAL
SYSTEM IS THE MAN WHICH IT
FORMS."

-HENRI FREDERIC AMIEL

DAY 175

"WHAT YOU PLANT NOW, YOU
WILL HARVEST LATER."

DAY 176

"IT IS A WISE FATHER WHO
KNOWS HIS CHILD."

-WILLIAM SHAKESPEARE

DAY 177

"LIFE IS TOO SHORT TO BE
LITTLE. MAN IS NEVER SO MANLY
AS WHEN HE FEELS DEEPLY, ACTS
BOLDLY, AND EXPRESSES
HIMSELF WITH FRANKNESS AND
WITH FERVOR."

-BENJAMIN DISRAELI

DAY 178

"TO BE A MAN IS, PRECISELY, TO BE RESPONSIBLE."

-ANTOINE DE SAINT-EXUPERY

DAY 179

"THE SEARCH AFTER THE GREAT
MEN IS THE DREAM OF YOUTH
AND THE MOST SERIOUS
OCCUPATION OF MANHOOD."

-RALPH WALDO EMERSON

DAY 180

"THINK LIKE A MAN OF ACTION. ACT LIKE A MAN OF THOUGHT."

-HENRI LOUIS BERGSON

DAY 181

"EVERY MOMENT AND EVERY
EVENT OF EVERY MAN'S LIFE
PLANTS SOMETHING IN HIS
SOUL."

-THOMAS MERTON

DAY 182

"WE DO NOT STOP EXERCISING
BECAUSE WE GROW OLD – WE
GROW OLD BECAUSE WE STOP
EXERCISING."

-DR. KENNETH COOPER

DAY 183

"LONG TERM CONSISTENCY
TRUMPS SHORT TERM
INTENSITY."

-BRUCE LEE

DAY 184

"IT IS BETTER TO STAND AND
FIGHT. IF YOU RUN, YOU'LL ONLY
DIE TIRED."

-VIKING SAYING

DAY 185

"YOUR BEST TEACHER IS YOUR
LAST MISTAKE."

DAY 186

"HERE IS THE MANLINESS OF
MANHOOD, THAT A MAN HAS A
GOOD REASON FOR WHAT HE
DOES, AND HAS A WILL IN DOING
IT."

-ALEXANDER MACLAREN

DAY 187

"YOU'VE GOT WHAT IT TAKES
BUT IT TAKES EVERYTHING
YOU'VE GOT."

DAY 188

"MAN IS LEAST HIMSELF WHEN HE TALKS IN HIS OWN PERSON. GIVE HIM A MASK AND HE WILL TELL YOU THE TRUTH."

-OSCAR WILDE

DAY 189

"FORGET FAILURE. FORGET
MISTAKES. FORGET EVERYTHING.
EXCEPT WHAT YOU'RE GOING TO
DO NOW. AND DO IT.

-LOU FERRIGNO

DAY 190

"SHOW ME A THOROUGHLY SATISFIED MAN AND I WILL SHOW YOU A FAILURE."

-THOMAS A. EDISON

DAY 191

"WE LIVE IN A FEMINIST AND
EFFEMINATE CULTURE. BECAUSE
OF THIS, AT BEST, AS A PEOPLE
WE ARE UNEASY WITH
MASCULINITY, AND WITH
INCREASING REGULARITY,
WHENEVER IT MANAGES TO
APPEAR SOMEHOW, WE CALL FOR
SOMEONE TO DO SOMETHING
ABOUT IT."

-DOUGLAS WILSON

DAY 192

"UNLESS YOU PUKE, FAINT, OR
DIE. YOU KEEP GOING."

DAY 193

THE TRUE SOLDIER FIGHTS NOT
BECAUSE HE HATES WHAT IS IN
FRONT OF HIM, BUT BECAUSE HE
LOVES WHAT IS BEHIND HIM.

-G.K CHESTERTON

DAY 194

"HAPPINESS IS NOT THE ABSENCE
OF PROBLEMS, BUT THE ABILITY
TO DEAL WITH THEM."

-STEVE MARABOLI

DAY 195

"YOUR STRONGEST MUSCLE AND
WORST ENEMY IS YOUR MIND.
TRAIN IT WELL."

DAY 196

"THE HAPPY LIFE IS REGARDED AS A LIFE IN CONFORMITY WITH VIRTUE."

DAY 197

"WHAT THE SUPERIOR MAN SEEKS
IS IN HIMSELF, WHAT THE SMALL
MAN SEEKS IS IN OTHERS."

-CONFUCIUS

DAY 198

"NEVER LET YOUR MEMORIES BE GREATER THAN YOUR DREAMS."

-DOUG IVESTER

DAY 199

"THE SMALL MAN GOSSIPS. THE AVERAGE MAN LETS HIM. THE GREAT MAN STAYS SILENT AND ALLOWS WHAT IS SAID OF HIM MAKE HIM GREATER STILL."

-STEPHEN MANSFIELD

DAY 200

"FATHERS ARE TO SONS, WHAT BLACKSMITHS ARE TO SWORDS."

DAY 201

"IT IS THE JOB OF THE BLACKSMITH NOT ONLY TO MAKE A SWORD BUT ALSO TO MAINTAIN ITS EDGE OF SHARPNESS. IT IS THE JOB OF THE FATHER TO KEEP HIS SON SHARP AND SAVE HIM FROM THE DULLNESS OF FOOLISHNESS. HE GIVES HIS SON THAT SHARP EDGE THROUGH DISCIPLINE."

-STEVE FARRAR

DAY 202

"I SPENT MY LIFE TRYING NOT TO
BE CARELESS. WOMEN AND
CHILDREN CAN BE CARELESS,
BUT NOT MEN."

-MARLON BRANDO

DAY 203

"YOU CAN FEEL AN EMOTION.
JUST DON'T FEEL THAT IT IS SO
IMPORTANT."

-JOHN CAGE

DAY 204

"THEN JOIN HAND IN HAND, BRAVE AMERICANS ALL! BY UNITING WE STAND, BY DIVIDING WE FALL."

-JOHN DICKINSON

DAY 205

"VIRTUE IS A STATE OF WAR, AND TO LIVE IN IT WE HAVE ALWAYS TO COMBAT WITH OURSELVES."

-JEAN JACQUES ROUSSEAU

DAY 206

"DEATH IS NOTHING, BUT TO LIVE
DEFEATED AND INGLORIOUS IS
TO DIE DAILY."

-NAPOLEON BONAPARTE

DAY 207

THE IRON NEVER LIES TO YOU.
YOU CAN WALK OUTSIDE AND
LISTEN TO ALL KINDS OF TALK,
GET TOLD THAT YOU'RE A GOD
OR A TOTAL BASTARD. THE IRON
WILL ALWAYS KICK YOU THE
REAL DEAL. THE IRON IS THE
GREAT REFERENCE POINT, THE
ALL-KNOWING PERSPECTIVE
GIVER. ALWAYS THERE LIKE A
BEACON IN THE PITCH BLACK. I
HAVE FOUND THE IRON TO BE MY
GREATEST FRIEND. IT NEVER
FREAKS OUT ON ME, NEVER RUNS.
FRIENDS MAY COME AND GO. BUT

TWO HUNDRED POUNDS IS
ALWAYS TWO HUNDRED POUNDS.

-HENRY ROLLINS

DAY 208

"THE MAN, WHOM I CALLED
DESERVING THE NAME

DAY 209

"GLORY GIVES HERSELF ONLY TO
THOSE WHO HAVE ALWAYS
DREAMED OF HER."

DAY 210

"AT TWENTY YEARS OF AGE THE
WILL REIGHS; AT THIRTY, THE
WIT; AND AT FORTY, THE
JUDGEMENT."

DAY 211

"MONEY COMES AND GOES, TIME
JUST GOES."

DAY 212

"ACCOMPLISHMENT WILL PROVE
TO BE A JOURNEY, NOT A
DESTINATION."

-DWIGHT D. EISENHOWER

DAY 213

"THE MEN WHO HAVE SUCCEEDED
ARE MEN WHO HAVE CHOSEN ONE
LINE AND STUCK TO IT."

-ANDREW CARNEGIE

DAY 214

"VISION WITHOUT ACTION IS A DAYDREAM. ACTION WITHOUT VISION IS A NIGHTMARE."

-JAPANESE PROVERB

DAY 215

"MEN ARE LIKE STEEL. WHEN
THEY LOSE THEIR TEMPER, THEY
LOSE THEIR WORTH."

DAY 216

"IN YOUR EVERY ENDEAVOR
REFLECT THE END."

-FRENCH PROVERB

DAY 217

"WE HAVE RESOLVED TO ENDURE
THE UNENDURABLE AND SUFFER
WHAT IS INSUFFERABLE."

- EMPEROR HIROHITO

DAY 218

"A MANS GOT TO HAVE A CODE, A CREED TO LIVE BY, NO MATTER HIS JOB."

-JOHN WAYNE

DAY 219

"BE SELECTIVE IN YOUR BATTLES,
SOMETIMES PEACE IS BETTER
THAN BEING RIGHT."

DAY 220

"VICTORY IS RESERVED FOR THOSE WILLING TO PAY ITS PRICE."

-SUN TZU

DAY 221

"DO WHAT YOU LOVE TO DO AND
YOU WILL NEVER WORK."

-CONFUCIOUS

DAY 222

"MAN CANNOT REMAKE HIMSELF
WITHOUT SUFFERING, FOR HE IS
BOTH THE MARBLE AND THE
SCULPTOR"

DAY 223

"THERE IS NO BETTER WAY TO FIGHT WEAKNESS THAN WITH STRENGTH. ONCE THE MIND AND BODY HAVE BEEN AWAKENED TO THEIR TRUE POTENTIAL, IT IS IMPOSSIBLE TO GO BACK."

-HENRY ROLLINS

DAY 224

"LEARN HOW TO LISTEN, AND
THOU SHALT PROFIT EVEN FROM
THOSE WHO SPEAK BADLY"

-PLUTARCH

DAY 225

"DO NOT SPOIL WHAT YOU HAVE
BY DESIRING WHAT YOU HAVE
NOT; REMEMBER THAT WHAT
YOU NOW HAVE WAS ONCE
AMONG THE THINGS YOU ONLY
HOPED FOR."

-EPICURUS

DAY 226

"THE ONLY TIME YOU SHOULD
EVER LOOK BACK IS TO SEE HOW
FAR YOU'VE COME."

"THE WORLD IS NOT LOOKING FOR SERVANTS, THERE ARE PLENTY OF THESE, BUT FOR MASTERS. MEN WHO FORM THEIR PURPOSES AND THEN CARRY THEM OUT, LET THE CONSEQUENCES BE WHAT THEY MAY."

-WOODROW WILSON

DAY 228

"WE AVOID RISKS IN LIFE SO WE MAY MAKE IT SAFELY TO DEATH."

DAY 229

"TREAT A MAN AS HE IS, AND HE WILL REMAIN AS HE IS. TREAT A MAN AS HE COULD BE, AND HE WEILL BECOME WHAT HE SHOULD BE."

-RALPH WALDO EMERSON

DAY 230

"DO SOMETHING TODAY THAT YOUR FUTURE SELF WILL THANK YOU FOR."

DAY 231

"FEAR IS PROOF OF A
DEGENERATE MIND."

-VIRGIL

DAY 232

"TO BE A GREAT CHAMPION, YOU MUST BELIEVE YOU ARE THE BEST, IF YOU'RE NOT, PRETEND YOU ARE."

-MUHAMMAD ALI

DAY 233

"GO TO THE BATTLEFIELD FIRMLY
CONFIDENT OF VICTORY AND
YOU WILL COME HOME WITH NO
WOUNDS WHATSOEVER."

-UESUGI KENSHIN

DAY 234

"THE PRESENT MOMENT IS FILLED
WITH HAPPINESS AND JOY. IF YOU
ARE ATTENTIVE, YOU WILL SEE
IT."

-THICH NHAT HANH

DAY 235

"TOO MANY PEOPLE SPEND
MONEY THEY EARNED...TO BUY
THINGS THEY DON'T WANT, TO
IMPRESS PEOPLE THEY DON'T
LIKE."

-WILL ROGERS

DAY 236

"IF A MAN ACHIEVES VICTORY OVER THIS BODY, WHO IN THE WORLD CAN EXERCISE POWER OVER HIM? HE WHO RULES HIMSELF RULES OVER THE WHOLE WORLD."

–VINOBA BHAVE

DAY 237

"A RIVER CUTS THROUGH A ROCK,
NOT BECAUSE OF ITS STRENGTH,
BUT BECAUSE OF ITS
PERSISTENCE."

DAY 238

"THE TRUTH IS FOUND WHEN MEN
ARE FREE TO PURSUE IT."

-FRANKLIN D. ROOSEVELT

DAY 239

"NO LOVE IS GREATER THAN THAT OF A FATHER FOR HIS SON."

DAY 240

"ALL MEN DREAM, BUT NOT EQUALLY. THOSE WHO DREAM BY NIGHT IN THE DUSTY RECESSES OF THEIR MINDS, WAKE IN THE DAY TO FIND THAT IT WAS VANITY; BUT THE DREAMERS OF THE DAY ARE DANGEROUS MEN, FOR THEY MAY ACT ON THEIR DREAMS WITH OPEN EYES, TO MAKE THEM POSSIBLE."

-T. E. LAWRENCE

DAY 241

"FORTUNE FAVORS THE BOLD."

-ROMAN PROVERB

DAY 242

"DUTY IS THE ESSENCE OF MANHOOD."

-GEORGE S. PATTON

DAY 243

"BRAVERY IS WAKING EVERY
MORNING TO FIGHT THE DEMONS
THAT LEFT YOU SO TIRED THE
NIGHT BEFORE."

DAY 244

"NO MAN IS ENTITLED TO THE
BLESSINGS OF FREEDOM UNLESS
HE BE VIGILANT IN ITS
PRESERVATION."

-GENERAL DOUGLAS MACARTHUR

DAY 245

"ALWAYS DO MORE THAN IS
REQUIRED OF YOU."

-GEORGE PATTON

DAY 246

"FIRST WE FORM HABITS, THEN
THEY FORM US. CONQUER YOUR
BAD HABITS OR THEY WILL
CONQUER YOU."

-ROB GILBERT

DAY 247

"IF WORK WERE SO PLEASANT,
THE RICH WOULD KEEP IT TO
THEMSELVES."

-MARK TWAIN

DAY 248

NEITHER A WISE NOR A BRAVE
MAN LIES DOWN ON THE TRACKS
OF HISTORY TO WAIT FOR THE
TRAIN OF THE FUTURE TO RUN
OVER HIM.

-DWIGHT D. EISENHOWER

DAY 249

"IT IS A HARD MAN WHO IS ONLY
JUST,

AND A SAD MAN WHO IS ONLY
WISE."

-GREGORY BENFORD

DAY 250

"HERE IS COURAGE, MANKIND'S FINEST POSSESSION. HERE IS THE NOBLEST PRIZE THAT A YOUNG MAN CAN ENDEAVOR TO OBTAIN."

-TYRTAEUS OF SPARTA

DAY 251

"MANHOOD IS PATIENCE.
MASTERY IS NINE TIME
PATIENCE."

DAY 252

"LICK THY WOUNDS AND TRY
AGAIN."

DAY 253

"IF YOUR SHIP DOESN'T COME IN,
SWIM OUT TO IT."

DAY 254

"NOW DOMESTICATION AND
SOPHISTICATION OF MEN BY
WOMEN ARE THE NORM AND
ACCEPTABLE BY SOCIETY, BUT
THEY ARE TERRIBLE FOR
MANHOOD."

-DEBASISH MRIDHA

DAY 255

"YOU WILL NEVER COME UP
AGAINST A GREATER ADVERSARY
THAN YOUR OWN POTENTIAL"

DAY 256

"CHOP YOUR OWN WOOD, AND IT
WILL WARM YOU TWICE."

DAY 257

"PEACE HATH HIGHER TESTS OF
MANHOOD THAN BATTLE EVER
KNEW."

-JOHN GREENLEAF WHITTIER

DAY 258

"PRIVATE AND PUBLIC LIFE ARE
SUBJECT TO THE SAME RULES.
TRUTH AND MANLINESS ARE TWO
QUALITIES THAT WILL CARRY
YOU THROUGHTHE WORLD MUCH
BETTER THAN POLICY OR TACT
OF EXPEDIENCY OR OTHER
WORDS THAT WERE DEVISED TO
CONCEAL A DEVIATION FROM A
STRAIGHT LINE."

-ROBERT E. LEE

DAY 259

"YOU BECOME A MAN NOT WHEN YOU REACH A VETAIN AGE, BUT WHEN YOU REACH A CERTAIN STATE OF MIND."

-HABEEB AKANDE

DAY 260

"CHARACTER IS HOW YOU TREAT THOSE WHO CAN DO NOTHING FOR YOU."

DAY 261

"MANHOOD IS DEFINED AND
DECIDED BY THE ABILITY TO
NURTURE AND TO PROTECT, BY
THE CAPABILITY TO PROVIDE
AND TO SUSTAIN."

-C. JOYBELL C.

DAY 262

"NO REST IS WORTH ANYTHING
UNLESS THE REST HAS BEEN
EARNED."

DAY 263

"A MAN WITHOUT ENEMIES IS A
DISHONEST MAN."

DAY 264

"IT'S NOT ABOUT HAVING TIME, IT'S ABOUT MAKING TIME."

"NEITHER IN THY ACTIONS BE
SLUGGISH, NOR IN THY
CONVERSATION WITHOUT
METHOD, NOR WANDERING IN
THY THOUGHTS, NOR LET THERE
BE IN THY SOUL INWARD
CONTENTION NOR EXTERNAL
EFFUSION, NOR IN LIFE BE SO
BUSY AS TO HAVE NO LEISURE."

--MARCUS AURELIUS

DAY 266

"THERE IS ONE RULE, ABOVE ALL
OTHERS, FOR BEING A MAN.
WHATEVER COMES, YOU FACE IT
ON YOUR FEET."

-ROBERT JORDAN

DAY 267

"DON'T LET YOUR HAPPINESS
DEPEND ON SOMETHING YOU
MAY LOSE."

C.S LEWIS

DAY 268

"DON'T BE AFRAID TO GIVE UP

THE GOOD TO GO FOR THE

GREAT."

-JOHN D. ROCKEFELLER

DAY 269

"BE STUBBORN ABOUT YOUR
GOALS AND FLEXIBLE ABOUT
YOUR METHODS."

DAY 270

"DISGRACEFUL, FOR THE SOUL TO GIVE UP WHEN THE BODY IS STILL GOING STRONG."

-MARCUS AURELIUS

DAY 271

"IN CHILDHOOD A FOOL THINKS ONLY ABOUT HIS FATHER AND MOTHER. IN HIS YOUTH, ONLY ABOUT HIS BELOVED. IN OLD AGE, ONLY ABOUT HIS OLD AGE. AND HE NEVER HAS TIME TO THINK ABOUT HIMSELF."

DAY 272

"ALL DARING AND COURAGE, I SAID, ALL IRON ENDURANCE OF MISFORTUNE, MAKE FOR A FINER, NOBLER TYPE OF MANHOOD."

DAY 273

"THIS IS THE TEST OF YOUR MANHOOD: HOW MUCH IS THERE LEFT IN YOU AFTER YOU HAVE LOST EVERYTHING OUTSIDE OF YOURSELF?"

-ORISON SWETT MARDEN

DAY 274

"WORKOUT. EAT WELL. SLEEP WELL. BE PATIENT. YOUR BODY WILL REWARD YOU."

DAY 275

'"OBEDIENCE TO LAWFUL
AUTHORITY IS THE FOUNDATION
OF A MANLY CHARACTER."

-ROBERT E. LEE

DAY 276

"YOU DON'T HAVE TO BE GREAT
TO START. BUT YOU HAVE TO
START TO BE GREAT."

-ZIG ZIGLAR

DAY 277

"HEROISM IS ENDURANCE FOR
ONE MOMENT MORE."

-GEORGE F. KENNAN

DAY 278

"THROW ME TO THE WOLVES AND
I SHALL RETURN LEADING THE
PACK."

DAY 279

"A LITTLE LESS COMPLAINT AND
WHINING, AND A LITTLE MORE
DOGGED WORK AND MANLY
STRIVING, WOULD DO US MORE
CREDIT THAN A THOUSAND CIVIL
RIGHTS BILLS."

-W. E. B. DU BOIS

DAY 280

"GO FORTH TO MEET THE
SHADOWY FUTURE WITHOUT
FEAR AND WITH A MANLY
HEART."

-HENRY WADSWORTH LONGFELLOW

DAY 281

"MEN ARE NOT BORN THEY ARE CREATED. POVERTY, DIFFICULTY, HEARTACHE, OPPRESSION, PAIN-THESE ARE THE THINGS THAT MAKE MEN OUT OF BOYS"

DAY 282

"AN INVESTMENT IN KNOWLEDGE
PAYS THE BEST INTEREST."

DAY 283

"LOOK NOT MOURNFULLY INTO THE PAST. IT COMES NOT BACK AGAIN."

-HENRY WADSWORTH LONGFELLOW

DAY 284

"A HAIRY BODY AND ARMS STIFF
WITH BIRSTLES, GIVE PROMISE OF
A MANLY SOUL."

-JUVENAL

DAY 285

"WE ARE WHAT WE REPEATEDLY
DO. EXCELLENCE THEN, IS NOT
AN ACT, BUT A HABIT"

-Aristotle

DAY 286

"ASK NOT FOR A LIGHTER
BURDEN, BUT FOR BROADER
SHOULDERS."

DAY 287

"THERE IS NOTHING MORE TO BE
ESTEEMED THAN A MANLY
FIRMNESS AND DECISION OF
CHARACTER."

-WILLIAM HAZLITT

DAY 288

ONE MAN WITH COURAGE MAKES
A MAJORITY.

-ANDREW JACKSON

DAY 289

"IT IS NOT MANLY TO TURN ONE'S
BACK ON FORTUNE."

-SENECA THE ELDER

DAY 290

"THE SMALLEST ACT OF
KINDNESS BEATS THE GRANDEST
OF INTENTIONS."

DAY 291

"A QUIET MAN IS A THINKING
MAN.

"A QUIET WOMAN IS USUALLY
MAD."

DAY 292

"NO ONE LOVES THE WARRIOR
UNTIL THE ENEMY IS AT THE
GATE."

DAY 293

"BY THE TIME A MAN REALIZES
HIS FATHER WAS RIGHT

HE HAS A SON WHO THINKS HE IS
WRONG"

-CHARLES WADSWORTH

DAY 294

"EITHER YOU RUN THE DAY OR
THE DAY RUNS YOU."

DAY 295

"BE STRONGER THAN YOUR
EXCUSES."

DAY 296

"NONE HAVE A HARDER FIGHT
THAN HE WHO IS STRIVING TO
OVERCOME HIMSELF."

DAY 297

"ONE DAY YOUR LIFE WILL FLASH BEFORE YOUR EYES.

MAKE SURE IT IS WORTH WATCHING."

DAY 298

"A MAN FINDS ROOM IN THE FEW
SQUARE INCHES OF THE FACE FOR
THE TRAITS OF ALL HIS
ANCESTORS;

FOR THE EXPRESSION OF ALL HIS
HISTORY AND HIS WANTS"

-RALPH WALDO EMERSON

DAY 299

"IF BOYS DON'T LEARN, MEN WON'T KNOW."

-DOUGLAS WILSON

DAY 300

"HOLDING ONTO ANGER IS LIKE
DRINKING POISON AND
EXPECTING THE OTHER PERSON
TO DIE."

-BUDDHA

DAY 301

"PRIDE COMES BEFORE THE FALL."

DAY 302

"LIFE DOESN'T GIVE YOU WHAT
YOU WANT

IT GIVES YOU WHAT YOU
DESERVE."

DAY 303

"ALL THAT ANGER. ALL THAT
FEAR. ALL THAT NEGATIVE
ENERGY, TAKE IT TO THE GYM
AND SPEND IT THERE. THESE
THINGS MAKE GREAT FUEL. LET
THEM NOURISH YOU AND NOT
THE OTHER WAY AROUND."

DAY 304

"'TO FORGET ONE'S ANCESTORS IS TO BE A TREE WITHOUT ROOTS.'"

"HAST THOU REASON? I HAVE.
WHY THEN DOST NOT THOU USE
IT? FOR IF THIS DOES ITS OWN
WORK, WHAT ELSE DOST THOU
WISH?

-MARCUS AURELIUS

DAY 306

"THE DEVIL DOES NOT COME
DRESS IN A RED CAPE WITH
POINTY HORNS, HE COMES AS
EVERYTHING YOU'VE EVER
WISHED FOR."

-TUCKER MAX

DAY 307

"IF UNWILLING TO RISE IN THE MORNING, SAY TO THYSELF,

"I AWAKE TO DO THE WORK OF A MAN."

-MARCUS AURELIUS

DAY 308

"IT IS BETTER TO LIVE ONE DAY
AS A LION, THAN A THOUSAND
DAYS AS A LAMB"

-Roman Proverb

DAY 309

"WE NEED THE IRON QUALITIES
THAT GO WITH TRUE MANHOOD.
WE NEED THE POSITIVE VIRTUES
OF RESOLUTION, OF COURAGE, OF
INDOMITABLE WILL, OF POWER
TO DO WITHOUT SHIRKING THE
ROUGH WORK THAT MUST
ALWAYS BE DONE."

-THEODORE ROOSEVELT

DAY 310

"GENIUS IS THE POWER OF CARRYING THE FEELINGS OF CHILDHOOD INTO THE POWERS OF MANHOOD."

-SAMUEL TAYLOR COLERIDGE

DAY 311

"YOU HAVE TO BE A MAN BEFORE
YOU CAN BE A GENTLEMAN."

-JOHN WAYNE

DAY 312

"TO BE A MAN REQUIRES THAT YOU ACCEPT EVERYTHING LIFE HAS TO GIVE YOU, BEGINNING WITH YOUR OWN NAME."

-BURL IVES

DAY 313

"OPPOSITION IS WHAT WE WANT
AND MUST HAVE, TO BE GOOD
FOR ANYTHING. HARDSHIP IS THE
NATIVE SOIL OF MANHOOD AND
SELF-RELIANCE."

-JOHN NEAL

DAY 314

"I KNOW NOT WHAT COURSE OTHERS MAY TAKE, BUT AS FOR ME, GIVE ME LIBERTY OR GIVE ME DEATH!"

-PATRICK HENRY, SPEECH IN THE VIRGINIA CONVENTION, 1775

DAY 315

"PRIDE AND EXCESS BRING
DISASTER FOR MAN."

-XUN ZI

DAY 316

"COURAGE IS NOT THE ABSENCE OF FEAR, IT IS THE ABILITY TO ACT IN THE PRESENCE OF FEAR."

DAY 317

"BE A WARRIOR NOT A WORRIER."

DAY 318

"THE MORE YOU SWEAT IN PRACTICE, THE LESS YOU BLEED IN BATTLE."

DAY 319

"YOU CAN PLAN YOUR WORK,
NOT LIFE.

"BE ALWAYS READY TO FACE
UNPLANNED EVENTS."

DAY 320

"FORTUNE FAVORS THE BOLD."

-ROMAN PROVERB

DAY 321

"THE GODS ENVY US. THEY ENVY US BECAUSE WE ARE MORTAL, BECAUSE ANY MOMENT MAY BE OUR LAST. EVERYTHING IS MORE BEAUTIFUL BECAUSE WE'RE DOOMED. YOU WILL NEVER BE LOVELIER THAN YOU ARE NOW. WE WILL NEVER BE HERE AGAIN."

-HOMER

DAY 322

"NO MAN STANDS SO TALL AS HE
WHO STOPS TO HELP A CHILD."

DAY 323

"EITHER FIND A WAY,

OR MAKE ONE"

- HANNIBAL BARCA

DAY 324

"FAILURE WILL NOT OVERCOME
ME, SO LONG AS MY WILL TO
SUCCEED IS STRONGER"

DAY 325

"TO THE BRAVE A FEW WORDS
ARE AS GOOD AS MANY."

-HIPPOCRATES

DAY 326

"IT'S BETTER TO DIE ON YOUR
FEET THAN TO LIVE ON YOUR
KNEES."

-EMILIANO ZAPATA

DAY 327

"THE BRAVE DIE NEVER, THOUGH THEY SLEEP IN DUST: THEIR COURAGE NERVES A THOUSAND LIVING MEN."

–MINOT J. SAVAGE

DAY 328

"THE TWO MOST POWERFUL
WARRIORS ARE PATIENCE AND
TIME."

-LEO TOLSTOY

DAY 329

"FIRE IS THE TEST OF GOLD;
ADVERSITY, OF STRONG MEN."

-SENECA

DAY 330

"ONLY THE WISEST AND
STUPIDEST OF MEN NEVER
CHANGE."

-CONFUCIUS

"DO THE THINGS EXTERNAL
WHICH FALL UPON THEE
DISTRACT THEE? GIVE THYSELF
TIME TO LEARN SOMETHING NEW
AND GOOD, AND CEASE TO BE
WHIRLED AROUND. BUT THEN
THOU MUST ALSO AVOID BEING
CARRIED ABOUT THE OTHER
WAY. FOR THOSE TOO ARE
TRIFLERS WHO HAVE WEARIED
THEMSELVES IN LIFE BY THEIR
ACTIVITY, AND YET HAVE NO
OBJECT TO WHICH TO DIRECT
EVERY MOVEMENT, AND, IN A
WORD, ALL THEIR THOUGHTS."

-MARCUS AURELIUS

DAY 332

IT IS A SWEET AND SEEMLY
THING TO DIE FOR ONE'S
COUNTRY.

- HORACE

DAY 333

"THERE IS ONE THING, TOO, IN WHICH THE WISE MAN ACTUALLY SURPASSES ANY GOD: A GOD HAS NATURE TO THANK FOR HIS IMMUNITY FROM FEAR, WHILE THE WISE MAN CAN THANK HIS OWN EFFORTS FOR THIS. LOOK AT THAT AS AN ACHIEVEMENT, TO HAVE ALL THE FRAILTY OF A HUMAN BEING AND ALL THE FREEDOM FROM CARE OF A GOD."

-SENECA

DAY 334

"NEVER TOO OLD, NEVER TOO
LATE, NEVER TOO BAD, NEVER
TOO SICK TO START FROM
SCRATCH ONCE AGAIN."

-BIKRAM CHOUDHURY

DAY 335

"MAN CANNOT DISCOVER NEW OCEANS UNLESS HE HAS THE COURAGE TO LOSE SIGHT OF THE SHORE."

-ANDRE GIDE

DAY 336

"DO NOT SEEK TO FOLLOW IN THE
FOOTSTEPS OF THE WISE. SEEK
WHAT THEY SOUGHT."

-MATSUO BASHO

DAY 337

"GET YOUR REST. MUSCLES ARE TORN IN THE GYM. FED IN THE KITCHEN. BUILT IN THE BED."

DAY 338

"SOMETIMES A MAN NEEDS TO
BREAK, IN ORDER TO
UNDERSTAND WHY HE MUST
NEVER BE BROKEN."

DAY 339

"ALL GLORY COMES FROM DARING TO BEGIN."

-EUGENE F. WARE

DAY 340

"THE SUCCESSFUL WARRIOR IS THE AVERAGE MAN, WITH LASER-LIKE FOCUS."

-BRUCE LEE

DAY 341

"DO WHAT THY MANHOOD BIDS
THEE DO FROM NONE BUT SELF
EXPECT APPLAUSE; HE NOBLEST
LIVES AND NOBLEST DIES WHO
MAKES AND KEEPS HIS SELF-
MADE LAWS."

-RICHARD FRANCIS BARTON

DAY 342

"FORGET WHAT HURT YOU, BUT NEVER FORGET WHAT IT TAUGHT YOU."

DAY 343

ANYTHING YOU DO CAN GET YOU
KILLED, INCLUDING NOTHING.

DAY 344

"BE PATIENT IN A MOMENT OF
ANGER AND YOU WILL ESCAPE
ONE HUNDRED DAYS OF
SORROW."

-CHINESE PROVERB

DAY 345

"THE RESISTANCE THAT YOU
FIGHT PHYSICALLY IN THE GYM
AND THE RESISTANCE THAT YOU
FIGHT IN LIFE CAN ONLY BUILD A
STRONG CHARACTER."

-ARNOLD SCHWARZENEGGER

DAY 346

"THE OBSTACLE IS THE PATH."

-ZEN PROVERB

DAY 347

"IF I WERE TO WISH FOR ANYTHING, I SHOULD NOT WISH FOR WEALTH AND POWER, BUT FOR THE PASSIONATE SENSE OF THE POTENTIAL, FOR THE EYE WHICH, EVER YOUNG AND ARDENT, SEES THE POSSIBLE. PLEASURE DISAPPOINTS, POSSIBILITY NEVER. AND WHAT WINE IS SO SPARKLING, WHAT SO FRAGRANT, WHAT SO INTOXICATING, AS POSSIBILITY!"

DAY 348

"CONTEMPORARIES APPRECIATE
THE MAN RATHER THAN THE
MERIT, BUT POSTERITY WILL
REGARD THE MERIT RATHER
THAN THE MAN."

-CHARLES CALEB COLTON

DAY 349

"NO MATTER WHAT HAPPENS IN YOUR LIFE, EVEN IF YOU LOSE EVERYONE AND EVERYTHING, YOU WILL ALWAYS TAKE ONE THING FROM IT ALL; KNOWLEDGE. AND WITH THAT, YOU CAN BUILD YOUR LIFE ANEW."

DAY 350

"SEE WITHOUT LOOKING. HEAR WITHOUT LISTENING. BREATHE WITHOUT ASKING"

-W. H. ANDEN

DAY 351

"IT IS NOT WHAT HE HAS, OR
EVEN WHAT HE DOES WHICH
EXPRESSES THE WORTH OF A
MAN, BUT WHAT HE IS."

-HENRI-FREDERIC AMIEL

DAY 352

TOIL AND RISK ARE THE PRICE OF
GLORY, BUT IT IS A LOVELY
THING TO LIVE WITH COURAGE
AND DIE LEAVING AN
EVERLASTING FAME.

-ALEXANDER THE GREAT

DAY 353

"MAN SUFFERS ONLY BECAUSE HE
TAKES SERIOUSLY, WHAT THE
GODS MADE FOR FUN."

-ALAN W. WATTS

DAY 354

"MASCULINITY IS NOT SOMETHING GIVEN TO YOU, BUT SOMETHING YOU GAN. AND YOU GAIN IT BY WINNING SMALL BATTLES WITH HONOR."

-NORMAN MAILER

DAY 355

"STRENGTH, COURAGE, MASTERY, AND HONOR ARE THE ALPHA VIRTUES OF MEN ALL OVER THE WORLD. THEY ARE THE FUNDAMENTAL VIRTUES OF MEN BECAUSE WITHOUT THEM, NO "HIGHER" VIRTUES CAN BE ENTERTAINED."

-JACK DONOVAN

DAY 356

MAN'S HIGHEST JOY IS IN
VICTORY: TO CONQUER ONE'S
ENEMIES; TO PURSUE THEM; TO
DEPRIVE THEM OF THEIR
POSSESSIONS; TO MAKE THEIR
BELOVED WEEP; TO RIDE ON
THEIR HORSES; AND TO EMBRACE
THEIR WIVES AND DAUGHTERS.

-GENGHIS KHAN

DAY 357

BRAVERY IS BEING THE ONLY
ONE WHO KNOWS YOU'RE
AFRAID.

- DAVID HACKWORTH

DAY 358

"A PROVERB IS ONE MAN'S WIT
AND ALL MEN'S WISDOM."

-LORD JOHN RUSSELL

DAY 359

"WE MUST ALL HANG TOGETHER,
OR ASSUREDLY WE SHALL ALL
HANG SEPARATELY."

-BENJAMIN FRANKLIN

"A MALE WAS TRANSFORMED INTO A MAN BY THE WILLFUL EXPENDITURE OF ENERGY. ABOVE ALL, A MAN WILLED HIMSELF TO BE EXPENDABLE. LIKE THE SUN, A MAN FED THE FIRE OF HIS HONOR ON HIS OWN SUBSTANCE. THE *MAGNUS ANIMUS*, THE *ANIMUS VIRILIS*, SQUANDERED ITSELF IN CONTEMPT OF ITS OWN DEAR LIFE."

–CARLIN A. BARTON

DAY 361

"HE WHO KNOWS WHEN HE CAN
FIGHT AND WHEN HE CANNOT
WILL BE VICTORIOUS."

-SUN TZU

DAY 362

"WE WILL BE RIGHT, OR WE WILL BE WRONG AND STRONG." (A drill sergeant warning his troops about messing up.)

DAY 363

SMALL BOYS BECOME BIG MEN THROUGH THE INFLUENCE OF BIG MEN WHO CARE ABOUT SMALL BOYS.

DAY 364

"THERE ARE ONLY TWO TYPES OF
WARRIORS IN THIS WORLD.
THOSE THAT SERVE TYRANTS
AND THOSE THAT SERVE FREE
MEN"

-SPECIAL FORCES NCO STEFAN MAZAK

DAY 365

"I KNOW NOT WHAT COURSE
OTHERS MAY TAKE, BUT AS FOR
ME, GIVE ME LIBERTY OR GIVE
ME DEATH!"

**-PATRICK HENRY, SPEECH IN THE
VIRGINIA CONVENTION, 1775**

THE END

67991330R00208

Made in the USA
San Bernardino, CA
28 January 2018